SUSAN BLANSHARD

POEMS FROM THE ALLEY

PAGE ADDIE PRESS
UNITED KINGDOM

CONTENTS

NOCTURNES

In the morning of altered ways
white blossoms lasting longer
if I return, to you, my lover
the fragrance will be stronger

whatever is loved, becomes a blessing
brings in morning, as milk
mixes with ashes, for alms—
as the pearl-bowl is lowered

whatever exists in a place, and so on
a place on grave mound found
a long line of otherworld ghosts
gather winter sedge in timely mist

each face with familiar features exist
in former times more than beautiful
The Lovely Ones, wild and licentious
decline with the seasons, to become
an auspicious collection of bones
kept under the old moon, I saw it happen
though I wish, not to grow old
all women's faces, gone centuries pale
but the reflection in the mirror—
was my-own orphaned shadow.

THE MONKS' GARDEN

At Ho Bo De Lake House
people come to pray for fortune
where bamboo grows, orchids open
a lotus is that, and lucky as well

there, fountain of moss and brick
beyond this, across the mist flowers
Temple Monks' left or fled, gone—
open, the lacquer gate

and gone, vanished silent
a thousand prayers come undone
it was strange emptiness, left eerie silence—
as an untended garden outgrows its despondency

yesterday, a drop of dew, sylvan by nature
handful of spice, incense or ashes, to catch
the slightest puff of prevalent wind
still gold-winged dragonflies appear a whisper
blossoms of apricot, peach gold and silver
on the same tree, defying verdant alchemy

we came here, in the same garden—
trees appear far and hazy
and forsake; branch, twig, leaves, the flesh
lucid seed, into a garden of floating light
between mirage and ghost—just where we chance
there falls an ever-after-shadow.

Out Of Sight

Now that your road is mine
its unlimited length of dust
the blinding plains of night
to keep your eyes from my face

rare stones, blue fires of fate
the exact moment hypnotized
I have absorbed the thirsty core
and what is more

I have already described
the muscle and bone of raw
feeling, the reason I undress in a hurry
and cannot leave this Lover

love of the road the blinding arias
stitched with sand and dust
saying yes, lead me to your body
by simple branch of yew tree

and the filigree of night
held the ancient coin
the blackened one they toss back
and it lands on the road
the face looking up
the same as the night
all silver bells—
my sight is yours.

The Memory Garden

In dreams a butterfly—still, seeking blossoms

A place of refuge is not complete
without a perpetual ally, to ask
is it better to be friends with Kings'
or with the butterflies

Nothing belongs to us, impossible this
request for a bit of earth, bequeath
I was only an ordinary gardener
and they wouldn't take it from a gardener

I lift my hand to a butterfly in the blossom
I found it myself, by chance
after a thousand things forgotten
I count everything I know—so

The butterfly effect changes margins
dissolves and vanishes in a moment
the garden becomes a kind of kingdom
in a leaf, a tiny boat

Two years of prayer has transformed
small sculptures and marble carvings
in merciful garden, a thousand years pass
it will be the making of us, you will see

Calligraphy straight as hanging needles
like lightning flashing or falling rocks
and infinite marks around raindrops
some as infinite as clouds possibilities

There are seven ponds of pink lotus—
it will be the saving of us, you will see
seven bridges over winsome water
when a thousand crane-birds fly
how the dead are carried directionally

Near or far in the eye of memory
something hidden in what you see
until the mind wakes with a question
still an insider in my own garden—
you should know that lovers are still here

I have looked at the rubric
why couldn't I have found this before?
you the butterfly—I, Basho's dreaming heart.

THE WATER CLOCK

It was in the season of eternity

Fishing in auspicious light
in blackened boat of buffalo dung
painted *fish-hawk* on the prow
strong in water, not afraid of wind
our oars bend endless water—
memory makes me remember
the lake wears more than one face

We catch fish east of *The Temple*
by evening, trap carp in west estuary
set our net where tide is deepest
like silk awash in the stream
among the drifting duckweed

Raindrops drip like newborn pearls
from green velvet leaves of longevity
and carp with golden scales
as large as our hands, as we passed
turns pond golden, pure and mystical

By the time misted rain falls, incarnadine
incense from the far pagoda
borrow sandalwood for sweetest dusk—
you and I watch smoke-wisps through sky
and before incense turns to ashes—prayers begin

Through and through, you understood by my heart
wild herons come with the season, as fragments
painted on a wedding screen.

Bo De Lake House

It is the season of crimson persimmon
birth of lunar moon, red and beautiful
like a sun-burned peach, gone ripe after rain

just a place for night sky to hook one moon
above the lake, more than single memory
seeds a thought of quantum destinies

there is dynasty, a touch of dragon that they swear
there is a feeling, luck resembles, to mark a new year
there is a surface, singular and simple, I have seen it—

and here like temple lantern all the moons are circles
there is song and reminiscence, looked and overlooked
any chancy moment, either it works, or it doesn't

the hardest thing, to weep in wind
or write a word in rain or sand, simply to be
to those who interfere with perfect histories

words worn-out, more than the oldest moon
lost in translation, or trifled hours—
it's a re-arrangement by *The Printmaker*

now, last cooking fire gone out in the old streets
much as horoscope's prediction, reckoning days
Master Dragon-Tamer has fled the world

years once lived by the flag's crude cloth
they remain, forever foreigners here
close the door on belonging—
and pass back the key.

THE BOWL

This, was here

A set of small bowls
Nestle inside each other
Double skin of red—
Lacquered wood
Easily held in the hand

In the art of placement
As the Monk said
When things look right
They feel right

The largest bowl for rice
The next for river fish
The next for vegetables
The smallest for sauce

In the art of placement
The Monk said
When things feel right
They look right

In the art of placement
Too many triangles
Triangles mean danger
So, they set up a tank
With six black fish—

Then hung up a red clock
Behind The Abyss
How would you guess that I
Should know rules, like this?
The Monk said

Others before you
Also went begging for rice
Begging for food
Everywhere, the rice grows
And the green fades away
All days go the same way
One by one, from time to time
As a game of mahjong—
The Monk said.

THE SLEEPERS

In a foreign landscape we are ghosts;
Entering the nights séance—

Capture what is still unaccounted
Immigration beads, flags of paper
Still swathed in wax seal and twine
They speak to us through deeds
In dust there are everlasting notes
You smell them on the old streets
One explosion after another
To draw you out of existence

I show you blood on my lip,
But this dried quickly
Resembles salt of memory and desire
You were my promise
Lips that gave everything
As your mouth moving across my body
And warmth presiding over

How we gathered our child
Second pilgrim of cold: enter dead land
As they send mysterious chill
Some shelter stolen one morning

Some you hide, others hate you
Use you until they change us

Like gunpowder
The black, exists so you can taste it
Just a bowl of burned rice
Or was it *The Cave* offering a place
In the silent stones
To sleep on the rough earth
Pulling the ground around you
What does it mean to sleep—
like a dog without a blanket.

FRAGMENT OF DAY

Then, far from The Paris of the East—
a collection of misted villages

in crowded market or opulent avenue
they chop down flowering blossom
and burn apricot limbs as fuel

now all songbirds have scattered
no one to cheer the lost-hearted
brambles fill the bereavement hall

to precede holly or mistletoe
mascara streaked, where shall they go
to open eyes and see the familiar

darkening skies full of snow flowers
phoenix mirror, unlucky broken
to conceal away with friends

as though ringed apart from cities
house after house, golden staircase
vermilion gate, neighborhood dogs

jade horses, flashing hawks—silent garden
seen through the bamboo blind
fragility forms a simple patent
but hardly possible—they will be here again

if we leave in the morning, we arrive at night
and in cold light outside the old house
what if, red lanterns where left alight—
we stay, in the quiet without a sound.

THREE BIRDS

Last night, thoughts within a dream
the water full of purple lotus

Seemed again, a great-leafed tree
Tall as the eye could see
To reach into the firmament

And the peacock in a silver nutmeg tree
With it tail long golden threads
Appears on moonlight branches

A bird of paradise, filigree light feathers
Had color of fallen snow

But then there was still white crane bird
It flies up into the red-blossomed cashew tree
Still with many feathers and quite unruly

Peacock-fan to adorn an ornate hat
Bird of paradise for a glamorous bower
Silk blind embroidered with dragonflies

Fabric and feathers go faded, even the butterflies
Turn gray, as color of moth
And the silkworm loses its bloom

Worn out, wasted, like all these things
And as before, regret locked in the storied room
Look back to follow birds over the snow clouds
Too soon, too soon;
Within the dream of the present life
There is a world of loss and poverty—
Return now the three birds: of luck, love and longevity.

ONE MOMENT

As far as eyes can see

A thousand books from the homeland
Something will be remembered—anything
From a distance, to hear falling waves
Head on silk pillow, to hear weight of ocean

And here, the sea at the edge of the island
Heat dampens summer clothes, sun's perpetual fever
What does it ever matter, if hair turns white
We are not young, we are not yet old

Whether happy, or not, whether good or bad
The broken heart beats with its own weight
A smile more valuable, they say, memorable
Lips smooth as marble Michelangelo's

As if, the *Master of Fate* knows what goes on
But on the thousandth night, we return
How long does a human life last
If no bed is left for The Perpetual Dreamers?

To enter this house without forging a key
Eight or nine majestic rooms, a clay tile roof
Ingenious cicadas, crickets' hymnal above
Twig-full of plum by the open door
Palaces dragged to the edge of the world—
I think of you, but how you do know it?

Treading On Grass

A path beside old mango trees
leads to The Temple of Literature
bells and chanting in The Great Hall
golden carp amidst simple waterfall
and reflections of your face
I see in The Jade Pool

Noticed at once, your soldier's coat
I had no way to send a message
now I see that your clothes are heavy
loss of your blood, my brother
I will wash your shirt in two separate lakes
empty a tearful of thoughts, where are you now?

Tears merge with thousand sheets of rain
field-crows gather after secular fighting
it is you that has not come home
it was you who took the bullet

a mountain of jade came crashing down
a memorial to bury a million bones
a stone statue, overgrown with moss
it crumbles by itself, with no one looking

I think of you, but I can't see you
when night comes and snow presses down
bones of the brave crack in the wind

the sound gradually grows older
everything is done according to The Rites
but no one can say, where you are buried.

THE CROSSING

One bridge over The Red River
Gustave Eiffel's second masterpiece
reaches up and over mosses and grasses

a simple house in north village-yard
light rain remains on the light dust
all old streets, alleys, walls, stones

all ways, of clay tile roofs, home
there is no summer in cast-iron roses
we are housed between earth and sky

one season, the river floods
one season, the river goes dry

now, when you come to the bridge
we must make separation
and go out through thousand miles
cross the river of dead iron-grass
how smoke-flowers blurred over the river
splitting our world to fragments.

The Return

There was a clamor of gold in the hall
Stolen for the King; gold bands, gold signets
Amulets enameled, a golden-blue confusion
Enough to ward off a thousand evil eyes—
Save one; for all the rings of centuries, look up
Golden days, secrets, the further one goes
Far off, who could separate gold from misery
But the treasures, just come with empty hands
Round the golden cup; drunk in a phrase
Everything of value—a handclasp away

For wealth, they choose the Emperor's pattern
Familiar, like a mother's Chinese vase
Here, in the opulence of antique porcelain
Spring trees covered in apricot blossoms
Petal after petal, became best fruit
And here, like gold-leaf of gilded fancy
Awaken every faded memory, all old, all endless
When gone their way, like wild bees
The last, in the rushing years, cannot be found

To drink mountain-apricot's bittersweet
Keep bones from growing older
Inlaid memories, sweet on the tongue
Until everything said, is undone
Honey left thick in the wilds
But hives have no taskmaster
We could live two hundred years
A thousand bees to keep us company.

NINE HEAVENS

With Nine Heavens as witness
before jade pavilion stones
someone painted stars that night
tore patterns from mulberry paper—
before you were born, the loved one

an angel pulls on nights shirt
light robe of celestial fabric
bright moon pearl stones are seen
fireflies in the mason jar, light-beams strum
crane birds come, and infant, the loved one

inked shapes in a far piece of garden
flattened rice fields with mistral hand
there is not a moment to forget—
for you enter the world, as loved one

now the moon brings night in close, but still
once fragrant plants overgrown with weeds
in topiary garden of mulberry trees allegories
months pile up bayonets of yellow leaves

The Gatekeeper sent to open the portal
and remembers—bathing you in The Pool of Heaven
and carrying you here on the assuaging hip
To see you far off, as the child within—
a likeness of beginnings.

THE BODHI TREE

It was the silk-worm month
The baby left under the bodhi tree
Blanket of silk in sedge grass basket
A small cocoon in the temple garden

Early morning while orphans slept
Like so many stars, all night
A child born into the world
Seemed to be from faraway gods

Sending silver bells and musical stones
Roses burgeoning with pink petals
In ninth month, pure life comes
Like incense embraces the moon

To keep, to hold, not give away
Now the orphan girl is waking
She was the gift in silk-worm night
Face of sleeping child, just becoming

Now hair all white, won for the years
Assail of the traditional calendar
Rustling pages vague, and vast
Seemed to be from faraway gods
A wish to keep family in one place
Son and daughter, close to each other.

Paper Money

There are lakes in Bo De District
where women speak over water—
they are not ghosts, *I heard them*

to see women at lake's inlet
sharpen knife on stone-hard steps
kill rooster, or Mandarin duck

wash herbs in water's curving jade
crouching on lower steps, pounding of wash
they were wives and fighters, *I saw their cloth*

they were lovers, mothers, child-bearers
more blood, to color water's reflection
some empty of love, some full of regret

just when they speak, no pretense of happiness
to argue in the marketplace, stammer out
ten eggs smashed, doubly wasteful, doubly dubious
interrupts overmuch; conjecture in hall of food
how the fragrant and the rotten become confused.

JADE PAVILION

This garden of contemplation—
here with dragonflies, inter-circling
cellophane wings with tremulous patterns

Is it the wings that move
or wind, moving the wings
either way, panacea of days

Here, verdant moss grows on old stones
tiny sweet pea, pale green leaves
violet flowers, some boil for tea

The seed, from seed of destinies
found in a Haiku of Basho
on last day of natures' séance
jade pond fills with darker carp

The Knower of all emptiness and loss
fore-shadow's a wrecking-ball future
proof, every dead-weight discriminates
under flood-light glare, criminalities
to steal from the ground up, it's hard to forget

After midnight, trucks go beyond city limits
now, everywhere is brick-dust! Birds in dusty flight
longevity lost by machete or knife
defer a thousand things in the name of progress
but not this divine place—a garden is forever lost.

Paper Lantern

The lantern is made for you to continue
a little slower, yet a pattern well cut—
filigree configuration meshed like stars
to challenge; the sound of quieter folding

Through silence, all red paper lanterns
to make evening something, evenly
when match is struck and all moons hanging
over The Bridge of Prostitutes and Thieves
a thousand stars shine on the river—*but soldiers' come*

Lighted path, slow-moving road, leaves no track
where soldiers' bring the gun, no one told
but the war was over, either there is a war—*or none*
who will tell—new ghosts' in their wander
over old Bridge of Sanctions, must stay out—*unless*

There is lone star on a flag in a darker fashion
this extreme gold gave an impoverish pattern
but hold familiar lanterns of night, engraved
within, and seeing, not seen, lantern's gold
an answer to yes, or no, depending on interpretation
interpretations or interpretations interpreted

And no one knows—a flood of propaganda
could be darker than a woman's red lipstick
one voice conspires against the future, hear it
if all paper is torn, if the candle gone out
it breaks up golden light and steals a piece of heaven

Raise the red lantern, see if light is counterfeit
or, back to the light, pour jasmine tea
if answers sought in the bottom of a cup
and dead leaves grow stronger

Will waiting for luck, make luck empty—wonder
look towards one another
secrets flash, like yellow lanterns in sunbeams
but closed eyes—look again
there are lovers and lovers and lovers
here saying—*whisper it*—what comes next?

THE SPADE

In moonlight, a man digs with sextant's spade
beneath dense leaves, conceals The Crown of Jade
every tool, shovel, knife, axe, gun, carries with it
a signature, by which it has been created
freedom for some, when the digging stops,
time goes back, it's not as it was
leaves a mother's heart, disconsolate

They could not hear our children calling
they heard only the Viet soldiers'
return home from Marble Mountain
back to the village, 'Mother, come out the door'
put on powdery white, white cloth, before mirror
when the brother heard, lost ones are coming

Just lent, a hundred dung boats, but one simple oar
crossing The Red River, surge and splash
November borrows tomorrow's sorrow
now soldiers congregate in The Luminous Hall
red-grass and dirt, moth-worn blanket matted down

Everyone says it's wrong, to let soldiers' go
without proper send-off and goodbyes
enough mourning, to know this, infinite missing
when a thousand men are side-by-side
just how much the same they look

The red flag, how low it flies
with a red splash of rain and blood
somber incense burns melancholy dust
a shrine to reach *The Immortals*
who can tell the sound of lost voices
from the sigh of a grieving woman
she's thinking of no one at all
she's thinking of no one special
ask her what she's looking for
where bleached bones lie
unclaimed.

THE QUESTION

Before the sun goes down in Da Tuong Alley
Cooking-fires alight; night-air lotus incense
Confuse cinnamon with tamarind-smoke
Ghosts and Sages watch, speak of past

Yesterday, a hundred patriot bodies found
In the garden of *The Magistrate's Villa*
To ask a question is simple
Do you know where —your brother's bones?

To walk over a field, the simple act
Dreamed he'd again come back
Knew us, and all the jade pendants, for luck
Hair white as old jade, all that is left

In the ash-hour, ashes go where winds deem
As Tantalus jar and columns of jasmine
Out of the war, and land that dreamed
There's many an unknown soldier gone

He passed among fields of burning rice
No welcome sound in a stray bullet
Only shadow, in red flares refrain
The damp grass, that bright scarlet stain,
All blood is ruled by *The Arbitrator of Fate*

Having died has its advantage
Each bone sprinkled in immortal dust
Destined, they cannot be transplanted
Deep and old, they can hardly be moved
I look for my Father, but he stays behind
Time that passes away, never comes again.

OVERTURES

To travel from one city to another
before the last one, and this one
a country, a history, a foreigners' memory
of typhoon danger and burnished sun

when will these humid clouds lift
even a salted ocean wind dies hot
at night sleep under gauze net
with an audience of mosquitoes

no good dreams on the bamboo mat
toss and turn months away
no one will know, as fabrics grew thin
some voile entrapment ensues

crewel net of nothingness
who's to say, the found are not lost
between China Beach and the sea
nothing to be done, in a cheaper room
but now, then, drumming rain
strips jasmine of its earthly flower
fragrant carnage in the morning
fanning the path, under bare-feet
hot as the summer was.

THE PEOPLE'S PARK

Summer heat which seems infinite

Old wrought iron fence painted blue
Surrounds the People's Park
In the green lungs of the city
Gustave Eiffel's third masterpiece
In the golden days of merit
Mandala of the immortals on far pavilion
Made a sundial in the *Fu-sang Tree*
Marble angels dance in the putti fountain
Faces peer through cool roseate mist
Like small children glad to get wet
Buffalo girl and fishing-boy
Without a bamboo stick in hand
But a belief the wings of the waterfowl
Could lift with six feathers

A thousand miles, north and south
Beyond Nine Roads from The Old Gate
East and west along The Seven Paths
A shift of the city compass
The summer not over, by half
Heavy brocade of lotus leaves
Planted tomorrow, by *The Master*
Every bird kept up their song
A good summer knows its season
There are topiary aces and spades

Box tree hedges shaped like hearts
And diamonds, shaped by the gardener
Until there is nothing left to do, but gamble.

Bone Jar

Some choose to fill the myriad hives
with lotus honey and wax from joyful bees
therefore this sweetness and light
for familiar bones to be kept perfectly
everywhere earthenware honey pots
but now, when told where ghosts have gone
only the bamboo flute, its fipple song
for the mourners, as the river rises
and the forever lanterns are lit wisely
the year of the rat passes
before The Golden Ox
the year of the dog and cat
and year of bee, long before that

They were always there
the honeybees that follows
an echo of pollen left behind
who tells the rest with pleasure.

SONG BIRD

How much remains

East of the Art Deco apartment
Faded colonial architecture, high wall
Consulate buildings on embassy row
Splendid trees with enameled plaques
Identify the cardinal Latin names
Perhaps, the glories of avenues and park

Morning, a thousand songbirds
In a flight of city's compass
And return a hundred times
In the mahogany and aspen trees
High branches, splendid feathered canvas
Winter birds call back and forth

Swallows fly home, ducks wing south
Bird-hunters' take them from us
Songbirds safe from no one
Birds flew to higher branches, silently
Sunday, it was—a day of entrapment

They trap them with a little honey
They trap birds for a little money

At the market, doves and orioles
Captured, like oriental culprits

Soon there will be no other singer
First a thought, and then to escape
A broken lock, flash of yellow
Forgive the ones that do not sing
To make this song, the older one grow
Long and drawn out, sad as sorrow
In order to release tomorrows.

Night Roses

When the window is open to the garden

Lights of near-by houses were out
a thought of blue moon, slanting over sea
the night, soldiers broke the garden's filigree
conspirators under darkness, unleniently
trod over bones, search influential wealth
ransack gold and precious embroideries
broke familial estate taboo, by pen or gun
all that was corruptible became confused
as wild bees in a smokescreen

what if, the foreigner brings their own troubles
what if, the visionary Saints have given
the shrouds, carried beneath tired arms
two by twos, one by one, the regrets
gather histories, perpetual momentum
like a prayer, a hymn, a charter for the rich
blood-fortune accumulated, is dispossessed

it is like entering a cold grave's desolate void
leave richness, and warmth of material ways
dangerous legacy, they always say
do not carry valuables from older days
do not talk of more than tomorrow
hide-away from where you came originally
to live like an imposter: for only shame
please, send a letter an invitation back again.

ONE PIECE OF JADE

In this intrinsic life, wealth knows no end
when a mansion house came crashing down
they say, to be born with talent invites disaster

they did not sip wine, from The Tree of Misfortune
and then not thirsty, the shadowy soul
says too much love, makes *Fortuna* jealous

how a foreigner in occidental places
in the rank of women, when all is turning young
fortune kept its distance, and so now bartered

every day cheated by similar strangers
starting to eat, like one not starving
opium pipe full of smoke, like one not drowsy

all this coming and going, far and away
finish off all these things, but do not stay
still, those who dream most, as night is set

turnover true treasure, particular stones
washed in The Mountains of The Immortals
the bangle of old jade a Lover gave

for a while, in another time, as it was—
luck, life, love and all The Dragons' of Fortune
a wealth rare in this world
carry the message to the end of the river
with time in life left, it was never too late.

OF SMALL THINGS

Grasshopper flicks cellophane wings
Of both dark and green, nothing more
Under eaves, above the red door

Thoughts all over my mind
Like cicadas on the branches
Of the cinnamon bark tree

Some cannot forget a voice
And if they could, it would be
To throw the past away

For a moment a misted rain
On the jade-green lake
A solitary swan, pale and still
How it stopped singing
When it lost its life-long mate

Everything becomes fragile
To look at a handsome face
Not the same as it was
Contemplate this ulterior mirror
Hair white as old jade
The longer we stay here, the older we go.

THE FRANEURS

Every street is called by anecdotal name
mentioned in estranged histories
dreaming things that might long to be

slip away, must leave behind
precious home, among everlasting theorems
yet, able to see where everyone sat

to know each ghost, one thought
the mind plays implausible tricks
but it was a fault in faultier stars

past years cast peculiar shadows
and so, become The Franeurs
just to invent imaginary places

all enriched with gold ornaments
construct significant courtyards
timely alcoves, arcades, fountains

black velvet drapes obliquely analogous
as a black cat in the dark—if one looks
for luck, luckier than the vision

for the materialists of the outer life—
to source first editions, the first folio
paintings of Picasso, his ceramics also

re-share life's diversions
an amalgam of has and have not
she is rich, isn't she, and poor too

or was she just a wanton shadow
slept on dirt floor, uncomfortable
look at this house, see nothing Cinderella
if ruled by the prince of perception
there's a strong possibility, all of this is fake.

THE ALMOND TREE

Of the trees that came to be
In the courtyard of Maison Gaol
Through chinks of time—in near past

Human or inhumanly, impossible
Some men are taken by the gallows tree
With chromatic leaves overhead
Even after, even after

After red lanterns are lit
After lipstick red kiss
After jade's perfect luck

Some men are taken by the gallows tree
Near lotus in the mudded lake
After rain fell with the night
After shadower of sorrow

Before night woke tomorrows'
Birds will gather in familiar branches
What else to do on allegorical mornings
Not to embitter litanies of trouble

There are names etched on prison walls
There are soldiers of brinkmanship

Who will take you as the worm is turning
As birdsong dies beside the dying

Sharp echo of polished boots
Across rain wetted courtyard
Some men are taken by the gallows tree
Now birds in the tree have gone

One gardener rakes fallen leaves
The almond shell in two halves, to remember
The wood of a sacred cross
And the kernel food for a saint

After sweeping, collecting, this gathering
All age-lasting rust of the fallen—
Until the whole season is in his arms.

LOVERS' TREE

Some women are taken by The Lovers' Tree
with embroidered bower overhead
each wedding-crown and veil
even after, forever after
after candles are lit
after lipstick red kiss

lovers' use red, like spice
of all things beautiful, conspicuous
to you, to me, I know one thing
the kiss will taste like you again
will night wakes a thousand tomorrows'
love you forever, as light fade away

after pearls given for luck
after rain falls with the day
some women are taken by the lovers' tree
near red roses in conservatory
doves ever gather in familial branches
what can they do on allegorical day
but listen to Medici's Marriage Choir

There is a moment, like a dream
and this was, soft echo of wedding shoes
across the flagstones to the long-gate
some women are taken by The Lovers' Tree
now the love-letters in the world are collected

a poet holds the richest pages
The Embroiderer of Names, love is found
after the writing, collecting, the gathering
all age-lasting letters of *The Lovers*—
until I saw the whole season in her arms

Now, marriage flowers all fallen and gone
the nests in the branches belong to love-bird
even a sparrow has found a home
and the swallow a nest for himself.

TEN STEPS

The way home is close—
memories circle around, months pass
but thoughts of last summer, multiply
no one lives past a hundred, no one asks why

why not, ask this older woman,
she, ninety years, wears silk pants
inside out, and satin slippers in dirt

not for want or laziness, the gratitude
wear black, as clothes grew old
she whistles away, *The Thousand-Mile Song*

a woman goes where she wants to belong
to wash shirt and pants in two separate lakes
machete tied by rope at her waist
a knot that can't be loosened
just now, rain drenches darker cloth
an arrangement of women's blood

where it will cut, when knife goes through
green snake on dirt floor and sound of voices
aware of a soul, no-one can change

who can tell, if she old, or older
she has killed in her time—a soldier
yet once she coaxed a bullet

follows less instructions than inclinations
called back to the garden, by The Dead Men
perhaps, as she is now, in simple moments
The keeper of quieter histories

just look at the rusted gate—iron like willow
rainwater is softer than iron or lead
but lead will poison well-water

always urgent—today is gone tomorrow
sharpened knife on a block of stone
hope for a long life without a dire end
drink the wine, while the garden
grows more weeds than flowers.
and the gardeners are gone.

The Kite Maker

Open the red door—courtesy of the army

The King has ordered a holiday
For the pattern of righteousness

Whiskey jar and wine confiscated
Pure potable water, also

Once more, gun, bomb, and drone
Knows nothing of the Tao

Who shall know at the start
If the offering for luck

Is properly done, or not
A pattern is set, for ceremony

To see foreigners avoid discrepancy
After the nine to five curfew begins

Green rice cake and betel nut
Strong women, deeper thoughts

Light this silver pipe of opium
Flute and drum closer together

Bring out paper dragon kite

For good reasons, to send
Remembrance to far heavens

Wind will tie the sedge knot
Winds rise, Viet kites fly
Until the edge of blue-washed sky

Cast the string and send off
Hidden prayers, quieter histories
High and lucky, but parted from this

Red and sere, above the pavilion
And sure of meeting again
But then, the months grow long
The string grows loose

If you wish to die, there is no way
If you wish to live, you know not how
Just a parting and reunion
So, it's you, Lover at every crossing
A short step away, then I am young—
Who can think of no return.

SHUTTERS

All is rain, insentient and driven

tapestried properties and the bronze
bell of the Temple, deep baying
poverty must beg from providence

there were monks and novices chanting
stirring-up, song-lulled lotus world
and a poem of flowers as well
frangipani, sweet cassia, honeysuckle
punctuating immortal mornings

walking with the rain mist, stinging
eyes, shaping vulture turrets
of colonial mansions on Ly Thuong Kiet

shadows on the road to winter
the city spreads orange clay-tile roofs
so many people; lost as before

in a roomful of felicitous thought
silence then, silence slow
like a death, I have lost myself—
open the shutters, wider, wider.

FORAGERS

In the estate of the drug lord
side-yard of this mansion-house
legend says curious treasure is buried
gold doused by torch and bright moon
enough to pay a thousand years rent
between the old well and mango tree
so—watch the night

There were comings and goings
from the here and now
from dusk till dawn
day and night *The Foragers*
for some trifling reason
climbed the walls of the illusory

Like autumn leaves, green snake
they enter unlocked mansion gates
pillage the house, rifle rice sacks
until dirt features on a hundred hands
as though they sieved through the land, itself
to search for the imprudent year

There were other conspiracies of hierarchy
once distracted by a stranger's name
metal on four walls of the hiding place
also, disgorged lock-room, snowed cocaine

Starved on rice grass and artichoke tea
the monk sat next to the mandrake tree
invited the drugged ones to search again.

Pull up The Golden Curtain
I think of you, but you do not know it
and step out into the gilded day.

THE RED GATE

Halfway into the old city walls

An official measured-up iron fence
told us, a singleness of single purpose
random dead ducks 'We will clean up the filth'

No dogs, chickens warm-blooded things
unfit for consumption, as the market begins
pull down the two-hundred-year-old market
to put up a western-style supermarket

In The Old Quarter streets the noise deafening
red silk dragons passing by, men beating drums
and pounding gongs, the women dancing
silver pins in their jet-black hair

Tolerate noise, though sound is intolerable
the patriot ghosts are slow to arrive
in a moment, see crowds with funeral flags
black and white banners and the women crying

Inside a house in The Old Quarter
books from The Bookworm, where will they search
move the bed, disturb black-legged spiders
doors open into depth of patriot tunnel

worry, already anxious, under the regime
gun pointed in the face, careful
even a shadow is not safe on the wall
a single light behind the curtain's disarray

afraid of a trap, as more army arrive
words pointed like gun's bullets
trickier than propaganda's agenda
sparing of speech, only to stand there,
a statue forgets which face to put on

then a hundred shadows, darker than the dye
Moral police arrest you after midnight—
do not speak of this place again.

Song Of Gecko

Oh —the flag they will fly

Every day I think of you, my friend, my brother—
in the ceremony for the foreigner

There is something odd in the cul-de-sac
At the end of the road, more than you knew

The People's Army brought their trucks
And closed the local market down

Stalls upside down, guns in the shadows
A hundred people close their windows

Make beds like a shroud, as night comes
Without making an error, too many spies

Everything according to the rules
Everything according to the rites

Follow the principles, agree, no argument
Hostage to regicide and usurpation

A thousand bricks seal houses behind the wall
Sorry for the poor, nothing properly weathered

Air gone stale, now mold grows like black coral

Red lantern light attracts golden geckos

But soon blue walls turn to mildew
Lacks the fixity of now and forever

The rice is not harvested, how shall they eat
Know change won't wait—people grow sicker

Some took Chinese vaccines in the pandemic
Opium left milky silhouette, for quieter belief

Better to drink peach wine, and hide the wreath
Silver buried in the plot, but gold holds the future

A pint of rice costs ten pints of gold,
All passports confiscated by *The Giver of Sorrow*
To cross the world, no bridge from tomorrow
Unlucky year of the rat could get no worse

Every day I think of you, my friend, my brother
A traveler's heart—in the ceremony for the foreigner.

HANOI

A rented villa, views of the market
Painted walls, all its carved rosettes
Open the shutters and watch the women
Cutting catfish for rice fields, for daily soup

There are live dogs in cages, curly tailed
Flocks of songbirds in bamboo cages
Tangled notes add to the shrill and loud
Mynah birds and nightingales, singing
It sounds as if falling from the sky

Catch the scent of ginger and jasmine
A thousand miles beyond—I turn my head
The gates to *The Tamarind House* fly open

Who belongs to the inner room
Not having swept away nomadic dust
Restless selves that break the heart.

DEATH'S CRUDE PLUCK

They tore a white linen band
And tied it
Low, across your forehead

Your face whiter, shade of pale
Simple thin line where a smile is lost
The fallen cannot be gathered

You won't come back that day either
When you sleep through
Or, don't come home at all

Shout out your name
Such secret memories stay with me
Even as monks' strip bed bare

To look back and a true likeness
A vision of a handsome face
In the yin and yang mirror

But then, spurred away
Too fragile to endure the sound
Of flute and drum beat, discordant
As woodcutter nails planks
For a grandiose coffin

Moments kept company with the lonely

Barely withered lotus, and perished
Yellow roses in snow thaw, crumpled notes
Found in the last coat you wore
Shrapnel of spare coin, cold in the pocket

Nothing left to do but go
Hide in the greener place
Listen to rice grow

No one spoke of shadows
Silently, they join us
Lie down in the burial-field
One by one—
As if by example.

LIBRARY

Most people expect our journey, incredulous
To cover Far East in a thousand months
One country at the end of the road

Yet, we didn't know where we were heading
Or if, dead ashes can be ignited by fanning
A sense of resignation: let it burn!

As it may be paper, yet not paper
Worth less as a dead tree
To find where its book has gone

Last month, the illusions became many
Even *The Woodcut Dragon*, insentient
Pens and inking of a thousand years

Red stamp official seal, scissors and ribbon
For four hundred months, only to wish
Prayers for happenstance and fortune

Homage of paper, about to open
For the fortunate but still—where are
Passionate writings left behind by lovers?

WRITTEN

In the old capital city
flood waters receded
after the storm of centuries

on the way back home
the unfamiliar journey
to sit beside The Sword Lake

there was a canopy of willow
reaching down to touch
the calabash of green water
for no reason, each fallen frond

thin mist floats in the wind
chanting of monks emerge
through quiet moments of rain

see semi-golden face
immersed in gold thought
a monk's pure countenance

there is a white temple in Jade Lake
spring in the winter
blood in the Red River

a new moon that cannot be found
a moment in the Cochin rain
a caged song-bird in the sky
a small song of bamboo pipe

blessed with luck
while fleeing from disaster
to succeed in a great moment
unseen, some reason, no more than so

such as when the blind man
touched my eyes—somewhere
back in the Somerset countryside
to see a different the world
through the same eyes.

ON RENEWAL

Leave-taking is not easy
Multiple papers, red crossed ink
Then confuse lock-down situation
Find passport? A signature?

There has only been one place
In the world, so interminable
When a paper-trap is set
The stars shift positions

Surname is maiden name
Surname is married name
So, ask *The Master of Fate*
To send another fortune

Of the many soldiered road
Blood and earth at the end
Some would be shot for thought

There was a dossier on a desk
Of interest to the interested
Of the people, for the people
But then the people's people say
There is an army and ministers
As a rule, they are fathomless —
Like an empty boat pulled up on the sand.

The Foreigner

This land is not their home
But still, they come here
In the fourth and fifth months
When rice fields are greenest

A handful of rice; first of season
Bamboo basket, kept warm by cloth
Street corner, woman makes money
In a thousand ways, *I just saw her*

Opium scales held high in her hands
Divinely accurate, the weights summon
Red poppy and silken pod, like drunken ink
Tamed by the master's brush, it seems

Begging for rice, begging for food
Acres of lamenting heart
Lines of mascara tears;
Grateful a little narcotic residue
Let others eat green rice
And leave the ones, thankful to dream on
A silver pipe, a night of opium.

A NOTE

Silk strings on *t'ung wood*
Hush of bitterness and song
Sadly, sadly the moments are gone

As human shadows lengthen
As days blurred tomorrows
Blank pages in the book of sorrow
Once again *The Creator of Chaos*
Once you leave, you leave forever

But later, outside Hotel Metropole
Hoist red flag's semaphore of stars
As *The Master* raises his hand
In a bid for ordinary people to decipher

After five days of hot weather
The locals dream about rain
After three days of rain
They complain about drowning
The women standing at the crossroads
All women hugging their children
Things to let go
The wind helps me dry out tear-sodden books
Late summer on its way
And I am already dressed for winter.

MIDNIGHT MUSIC

Things are not what they seem
Art is a lie that made you recognize

There was a white picket fence
You could look through
If you wanted to
Possibilities look to be impossible

An Emperor who saw this
Stood there one summer evening
Took out the spaces with utmost care
And built a pagoda in the simple air

A white pagoda for his second wife
Clay-tiles like fractal dragons
Whimsical lanterns strung all over
A phantom only existing

Each fence post left there
With nothing around it—all objects
And no space more endless
And I wouldn't have seen it
On a blank sheet of white cloud
If I hadn't believed
One thing was certain
Sharing a common night and day
All of us, become truthful.

THE LEGEND

At Hoan Kiem Lake in long-fog
The heavenly ways of the Gods'
Treat one to heaven, on earth

Pink lotus flowers in pure water
A drop of water on a jade platter
A thousand lanterns, Red Lacquer
Bridge to The Faraway Pagoda

From somewhere a bamboo flute
Golden Turtle endures this, everydayness
With an edge against ancient histories

Heat and floods without death
Sacred sword in mouth, the legend
Is around—all this in keeping

Five times its golden head
Appears through pernicious weeds
See what is seen, foreshadows are rare

Everything is memory when it is gone
For luck?
Through the water again through lotus
Longevity sadly mortal
And in twenty or so years
The vision endures, the gift of time
Where would such turtle luck carry us?
See then, the luck!

BLESSING

The English foreigners are leaving
Burn paper horse for their journey
Bring in a red crystal ball

So the Monks' come early
How to perform a blessing
For borrowed, wasted days

And a small carved plinth
On this, the divination sits
By the weight of its own weight

Position it in the kitchen window
To realize how this is something
Of an anomaly, the reflection

From the lake, the sun catching
While small fishes fry
A bloody beam
Something will matter, even red flowers
Rice thrown to chickens

Those with tin eyes cannot see
In the courtyard they burn
A horse, shoes, several hats

A bundle of money and a jacket

Is it for the opposing dead
Those who have tin eyes

Paper and matches, or what?
To send a message, to guide a prayer
A sense of the necessity

See the incense smoke's godly path
Not black nor white either
Let it be a scent of dust and bone

It has a sense of purpose in the ether
Float in ink, float in wine
Let the bottle pour itself

Because, back and forth, no place to be
But in *The Kingdom of Hereafter*
Not every river has a worldly bridge
But I would give you a thousand boats
To sail back home.

RICE FIRES

End of summer, mercury high
Along the hem of highway
Rice fires burn the rice fields
Gleams of flame reach red moon
Flying embers fall into the stars
Reach beyond histories firmament

It has always been this way
It is the custom to burn the fields
For the new rice cultivation
White egrets among sprouted grain
Insects in bamboo hedges
Ducks in the lake of catfish

Chickens inside harvest threshold
Pecking at empty husks
In the New Year following
Peach and apricot blossoms

In blue & white Japanned pots
Each branch hung with red or gold
Packets with new dollar notes
Nothing is old, for the luck
Nothing is worn, as the oracles' deem

Then the sound of broken wood
Until the cooking fires are lit

Dig mud terraces, plant new rice
Tow the water buffalo and cart
The boy with a flute
The girl with a song
Riding on the buffalo's back
Where the water is deep, round ripples
And the fields of childhood, their golden pond.

UNCLE

Familiar man, sits on camphor-wood chair
inside the doorway, pours bitter tea
strenuous inertia, masterly inactivity

so little minutes make the days
little drops of water, little drops of sand
makes the ocean, makes the land

yet the simple act of human gesture
promise of a martyr, no cross, no crown
the actual Orient promised in miniature

where one bowl of green rice, was the same
and on and on this hunger's refrain
we have less or more, or part of it gone

but wise man saves the people
throws them coins and gratitude
keys of the rice fields and attitude

glass of noble, glass of poor
opium pipe, respite for dreams
what's more, what he believes, he becomes

who shows the ones to take full measure
break an old bridge to build another
gold washed from the palace gutter

light or shade of herbaceous temple garden
for all gold and silver above and below—
stand a little out of his shadow.

In Cities

The year 2020 almost overtaken
Year of the Rat, turned from luck
Into fatal plague; fever settles
Gambled and frozen, sanitize
The world's every living thing
While parks fill with numbered bodies

Beg money to buy a sterile mountain
Wash off germs' inscriptions
On the wall of evolution
Let them repeat this, long regret
Ten million people assailed by virus—
How anyone ever imagined this

Nine times out of ten
Unpredictable, perished
Probably, all the news to hear
Five vaccines proved safe
True or false, who truly knows?

Our beds faced each other
The sick body hurts all over
Air in the lungs, feels like a stranger
A murder of dusty-black ravens

Dreaming beyond lock-down world
Visitors are missing; life is about masks
Six astronauts left for Mars on Tuesday
While there is still a little room on earth
Head beyond the fields and garden
Brush off the dirt with white gloved hands.

LAMENTABLE

The moon over the houses of sugar workers
The pale magnolia tree as our neighbor

Empty hall and echo of cangues
But old feelings are secret: who can convey

Back in the painted house, again
Who loves; watch sail-boats in Shoal Bay

Every day, dream of white scruffy clouds
Rain needles on the kitchen window;

Alone in the house, Shoal Bay below
The edge of shore lies unbroken

Eyes take it in, but no one sees
Memory crowded with homeland, to no purpose—
Must one think of those responsible for this?

ANDAMAN

There is an old teak house
On the island of small elephants
It is like a poem, infinite blue waters

In a distance, no wave waits
Nor lei of frangipani around your neck
Nor to swim off the beach when full tide

Moon in perfumed florescence
To travel the distance, air of three skies
Ungloved hands, in the double-ness of things

Unmasked, a hundred colored prayer flags
Somewhere, the wood veranda, black dog marauds
Aftermath of monsoon, when high tide ran its course

Every night the sun dips into sepals of horizon
Red as blood, divining iron mountain
Immortal jungle, none will go there

So, we teach ourselves the otherness
Of the dragon boat, lucky ornaments
yellow flowers tied to the edifice

Follow sunrise, from one island to another
For all who make waves, face to face
Soon what matters of the past

To be in a place, where we are nothing
But the island-loving deserters
You make quieter histories

In faraway room behind the shutters
I see myself, keep hold of togetherness
Under lock and key's allegory
For what good is an island to me
All this, for you, that's the way it is
Unglove your winged fist.

MOUNTAIN WATER

So I always remember

We took a diversion in the road
Walked the riverbank track
Our small son between us

Between, an unstrained smile
As though we all belonged there

These things are past, half our years gone
No sooner here, than altogether gone

The crack of a tree stiffens branches
Hard black colors, gray-black, red-black

Only charred land of the mad fire
Overpowering smoky acrid

Whether we like it or not
Wind shifts the corpse of ash

The bones of a pet dog
Dormant in the curl of long grass

So much landscape, to us is grieving
Spoiled the ocher and emerald path

However far you wander
Your dreams cannot reach back home.

NEIGHBORHOOD

There is minimum of interference
If you sit with your back to the view

A foreigner on a crowded street
Must not watch the prisoner pass by

Or see his face, strangely swollen
Furtive glance, hubristic expressione

Do not ask the question
Or the nature of outcome

The bullet of measured surprise
How he looks, who he is

On each side of the prisoner's face
An inventory of emotions

Elimination at the point they depart
I saw a hand print in blood-stained grass

She showed me a map unfolded
In a matter-of-a-fact-way
As if no such day ever existed.

Oblique Shadow

When you have been somewhere
For a while, you earn the ability

To be, more, or less, invisible
Or escape into oblivion

Out-of-focus self-reflection, if you see
Mistakenly reversed without audience

You can't be sure you're on a journey
When you are lost in a crowd

Until our traveling eye converts
Birds into fish, the cities into islands

Gazing at these black mirrors
An alter ego, a spy on our actions

How others see us, away and beyond
Narcissus mirrored depths

Until the dog with a grin
Became the grin without a dog

The trees appear equally positioned
Sham trees creating orchards
Painted mockery

You see it, now you don't
There are shadows of imaginary lotus
Palm trees bend and be straight

The same ambiguities after the monsoon
The same visual paradox after the typhoon

Your kiss like a permanent signature—
I needed to know that I existed.

FOR BELLA

I heard black dog bark, in the deep ally
Fur arrow and swirls on its ridge-back
For the luck, but a black dog, they say
Walks through graveyards all night
Midnight, it wakes up the rooster
The bird heard, faintly praising the sun

But it was only the moon's bright pearl
Lighting up the garden—woke me
Then voices and incumbent footsteps
So the soldier from the north
Faced a gilded orange tree
An invitation to entered the house

I will offer you plum wine, to ferment
talk of fish, we piled up on the shore
A rusted hook on a bamboo-rod
Sometimes I wish I could ask for more
Follow you and try your fish-hook
A cascade of dollars, the sacrifice money

But our blood will never be broken
You leave, and I hear nothing more
And by his fallen steps, all he can do
Just open the door to our old garden
And whistle the black dog home.

SAIGON

Intone for the English foreigner

Bird droppings have dirtied
All the eaves and Buddha statues
Friday morning, waited for rice
From basket-seller on street corner

Pushed out of queue by local men
Brusque slight-of-hand, edgy glance
Across the street, a soldier with gun
But who shall follow the foreigner?

Secret police drink bitter tea
Black leather coats incognito
The uniformed knows the whereabouts
Take photographs of by deciduous oak

Or, imagine this is subterfuge
Like a broken clock only guesses time
When I left, what route I take
Whom I saw along the way

A lover, or drug dealer
Or, perhaps the winter rose seller?
There are notes to exchange by the way
Black market American dollars

Welcome gold shop's illegality
There is a sapphire to buy
From the government shop
Five karats and a slight flaw

All that belongs is known by *All*
Facet after facet, out of the blue
Flaws in every flawless life
Visible through *The Great Jeweler's* loupe.

ANOTHER DAY

Mai fills a wooden bucket with lime-flowers
to soak the day from her tired feet
in an opposite corner of occidental
water holds its edge, water turns
into a jade pond in temple garden
no sooner does her foot touch water

she sits down in quiet abstraction
beneath the water, all was silent
the jade and gold had vanished
her sadness grew sadder

someone throws down a pebble
water transforms into a small circle
which becomes a larger circle
which we cannot control

take water as a message, no one
lives in isolation, to see
the circle continues
to expand until it covers
the entire lake
there are ghosts throwing stones
ghosts listening, when someone is talking
and their voice becomes drowsy
turning vegetables into mint
silent burial of words, as soon as Mai speaks.

FAMILY ALTAR

And now, in The Old Quarter
Everything turns antique

Tell rhymers and reasoners
money discerned nothing saved
bygones, are bygones— no returns
as many befores as ever-afters
toing and froing, comings and goings
streets of memories, roads of blood
the path swept by finders and keepers
we walk away, losers and weepers
freedom is broke, blood asunder
nothing left of illustrious centuries
each beginning, has its unending
fat in the fry pan, dogs in the sty
quieter histories, in a blink of an eye
lightening hits maple, also, the oak
silence breaks the silences comeuppance
hear a sound, like human voices
as the soldiers' finale, footsteps away
who leaves no footprints of himself
bleached bones knew not, yours or mine
unburied, uncovered, scattered by war
now tracks are overgrown
too many ghosts at the end of the line.

The Tea Shop

The window is open; dog barks
constantly, I have sat in the kitchen
beyond the homage of silence

while women with stone mallet
crush river crab shells for red soup
there was a strange taste, somewhat mercurial

there was a sudden dragonish eclipse
fishes fluttered like silver leaves
filigree net held unspoke secrets

now, you and I, share unsettled times
foreign words wrought our lips
as we mute language born to us

as the bamboo flute needs a breath
regardless of this time in exile
I shall exhume all memories

I found a lifelong taste for you
your voice filtered in my throat
my lungs fill with the breath of you
fossils of our time
a palace of glass-fish bones—
breaking inside my heart

rain pressed down on bamboo branches—
one moment, we drink the river's soup
one moment, pack our bags and are gone
some things presume change

there are old villages, hidden by rivers
but you are the one who knocks on my door
to give me a winter coat, with magician's sleeves
but that was a long time ago.

HOUSE OF LEO

The moon in equinox, rose the tide
It was the time for new life, bring word

Hardest of all was simple birthing

Against brittle wood, fire, smoke—breathless
Moreover, ash and particulate in birthing room

Slip a mask the newborn while he is sleeping
Bitter bulletin of bush-fire season, smoke continues

More than that, everything known, will turn to dust
Indifferently, irreverent at this, fiery sarcophagus

The hollow-men, avarice bone-set
Cobbled wreath of maligned donations

Higher up, benevolence in black branches
Empty husks burst of energy

The savior saplings crush upwards
There and only there, all day long waiting
It's been twenty years already
Since you left, life will soon wear out.

New Year Visitor

Two women set the daily fire alight
in cold blanket of itinerant fog
as black dog returns late from bone yard
yesterday, when family ghosts
enter our house at midnight
invited or uninvited, they stay for a week.

So many years together in another sleep
floors swept and children prayed for
slay forlorn dirt and eternal dust
for ethereal visitors and their shadows
on the shiny surface, a visitor would say
the house seems, clean enough

and children appear, polite enough
only breath fogs up the articulate lens
no chance left to view a world through
who shoots a cat on a Monday
for killing a mouse on a Sunday
and so ghosts of soldiers, forlorn lovers

remain in alleyways and everywhere
such as before, more stories that follow
incense, cigarettes, opium on family alter
in high places there always will be
a distinct touch of impossibility
but now, instead of grenades, and wine.

THE METAMIRS

Less is more, providing one had more
They had little, and gained everything
Including what is not certain

Like a journey across quicksand
Back and forth until they disappear
Into infinities, like polished obsidian

It began with argot, a puff of smoke
In their faces—and the wallet was gone
The conspicuous inconspicuous

Or the inconspicuous, conspicuous
They could not be sure
But things merge into back-ground

Like a white-feathered bird
In the snow, lends allure
Or the devil's blossom

Masquerades as a flower or leafy twig
Untutored for the predatory,
And those who masquerade in the blind
Conjures up, hopes to outwit
The black merges with the dark pit
Men they knew, in effect, became chameleon
And so, a fortune goes.

Sleeping mat

But now—scent of summer
the heart longs
for a simple two-mat room:

I find myself falling
deep into your beautiful words
blurring my senses to everything
your voice magnetic
and all that is inside
I see the dream
between the words
saying yes
the remains of life we keep
all we have left belongs to us
inside another sleep—
night runs again.

FORTUNE'S SONG

Once they searched among fate's stars
and derive a natal horoscope
high roller number, woman of metal
could be a minister of communist party

rice for luck, birds of song
a golden sword of fortune
enough incense smoke to reach
paper kites sent prayers beyond
to keep the ancestors happy

then saw *The Golden Turtle*
raise his head through pernicious weeds
in such occidental moments
could talk the world away
when all about was unfamiliar

but now green rice is threshed
jasmine tea once poured gone cold
old black dog appears once more
all places that existed before
will exist without us there.

THE WEDDING PLANNER

The family complained, like ducks in a market
So bride-to-be does what is expected
Simply by saying yes to everything, 'I will marry'
Not even a smile, or a break in the tears
Strangely wedding gifts collect and show complications

Simply by saying yes to everything, 'I will marry'
Her parents' wish—Ah, there are letters of proposal
Strangely wedding gifts collect and show complications
The gold and the meat should not be together

Her parents' wish—Oh, many letters of proposal
There were the usual betel leaves, tea, pork, glutinous rice
The gold and the meat should not be together
New rice, green, if a large box is on the table

There were the usual betel leaves, tea, pork, glutinous rice
An equal number of square rice cakes
And here red silk sashes on the dresses
And a hundred paper kites lashed with red bamboo

She counts an equal number of square rice cakes
No appetite left, it is sadness that consumed her
Plates and dinner set of colored bone china
Where painted dragons appear to break loose

Many gifts wrapped in red paper
Solid gold, clothes, rice, wine, meat, and no coffee
A single fruit is doubtful, if sadness is the season
The moon in a red lacquer box, the Gods' know

There is a tarnished plan from birth, she resists
Everything, but now the past intertwines future
That women of former times, pawn their wedding clothes

Whiskey on his breath, one sharp word follows another
Frozen stars in matrimony's night
Crack in moon
Where luck slips out—!

Leave-Taking

Once, they tore up iron tram tracks
to make a million bullets

women burned valuable books
sold embroidered clothes for nothing

the rabbit caught in a trap with a tiger
but then, birds and cicadas tune up

fragrant incense rises like pencil marks
smoke uplifts from damp cooking fires

against the red silk sun, this firmament
see orchids, roses, as many weeping willow

knew streets older than the French names
white cursive script on blue tin signs
Ly Thuong Kiet Street, Da Tuong Alley—
everything pulls us back here.

PROTOCOL OF RICE

There are whales in a river of catfish
Their compass lost in muddied water
Each whale leans against each other
They cannot tell river from sea at all

Gone past, the fishermen
It's just the same as before
They move one's imagination
Who knows where?

Small fish on a hook dot the shoals
To make a deep-hidden spectacle of gold
Fish after fish, nothing more, nothing less
Let's stop the boat, this moment is over

Gone like passing duckweed
The lanterns are lit: the night black-pitch
Drift with away by morning tide
And the rain wets the soldier's coat

For fear, that on the fallen red water
There may still be a few drops of blood
How could anyone see them?

In years come and gone
To send off a single soldier
And families scattered by the war

Appear and disappear
Now fear, Red River bloodies forever

For years, a pattern of summer time
Burned blossoms and peach-leaves
And rice-burning season a month away
Sky and river are the same color

Burned clouds hold old rain
Rain on top of rain
Each drop comes like tempered knife
The clouds are never emptied
By memory of tomorrow's ash
In this travesty of river, and rain
The bait you hook is all the same.

Other Stories

So I remember Hanoi always

I look away and back again
Five years disbelief reigned
Those who know untold story

In fragments butterflies return
Especially out of envious, tall poppies
That tower over ever-scarlet sun

Emptying the safe of house-keeping
Before a downtown café opens
Talk a while, find a fistful of dollar bills

Perhaps thousands, you never counted
Passes like contraband out the door
With a French baguette and a cake

Half a kilo of coffee beans
Roasted in butter, taste like chocolate
Presently we spend money's envoy

A stove to replace the faulty one
A green glazed dinner set
From the poor man's pottery village

Silk blinds with butterflies

Embroidered in palest blue
Float when the breeze comes through

From the veranda you see
Dragonflies over the pond
A row of white birds, what lies beyond

Seeds of frost, a verge of words
Pins of rainfall, hard to come by
An arch of rainbow fragment

A poem of bamboo flute
Sees through all emptiness
We are expecting visitors

We sleep in the back room
Wondering what hour it is
Welcome two new pairs of shoes

To walk across green chill grass
Only brings back memories
Play the actor to suit the day
We spent all the contraband on you.

SHE

There is a shop in The Old Quarter
Where Thao sells her silk

The Blue Man came here
He was dressed in blue
The man with blue eyes
Bought fifty blue scarves—
Did you send him?

He and I, now traveling east
The snow is just as light as a feather
Our shoes make new footprints

No place in the world is safe
Or unsafe

Upstairs, wordless, the bed is warm
The bamboo blinds are drawn

Yesterday, I gave this man
Lingering perfume, the bluest cloth
But then I gave him, one thing
Unaccounted for

She gave the man on the silk-road
A flag of red with its one gold star
Blood of the motherland.

THE FRENCH QUARTER

All that woman wanted, men built
pounding, hammering overhead
narrow street, vertical stair case

there is a closeness to squalor
sight and sound to one other
intimate neighbors, sisters, brothers
put down a sedge mat and call it home

coiled and tangled, the roots of vine
betel vine grasps to hold old walls
trees-girdled in the storm drain
moss-bound crevices, tangled

heavy daub of voices, blot tranquility
 balconies draped with wet laundry
rivet my thoughts of leaving
in the contemplation of place

some are forbidden to belong
anonymous transient
merely, passers-by on the way
 to someplace else

invisible to the ones born here
families of ten or more
their glances skid over us

move, jostle, push aside
in a preoccupation to survive

all is heat and rain, insentient
trees-girdled in the storm drain
moss-bound crevices, tangled
betel vine grasp to hold old walls

tapestried properties and the bronze
bell of the temple, deep baying
there were monks and novices chanting
stir-up, song-lulled lotus world

sweet cassia, honeysuckle
punctuating immortal mornings
walking with the rain mist, stinging
eyes shaping vulture turrets
of colonial mansions on Ly Thuong Kiet

shadows on the road to winter
the city spreads orange clay-tile roofs
so many people; lost as you are
in a roomful of felicitous thought
silence then, silence slow
like a death, I have lost myself

open the shutters, wider, wider—

DA TUONG ALLEY

Night removed itself and morning came
Cluttered with fog, thick cold rain
A bean curd landscape they call it
When the fog and cloud lay in slabs
And the dawn and day meet each other
Crowds come into the alley
Like orchids, faces unfold and open
The women squatted down
In the vociferous din of the street
Shouting their way under round straw hats
The emotional structure the people
Large baskets of garlic and ginger
Bitter cucumber, chives and taro
Holding cups of hot green tea
The rice is ripening in the field
Harvest is due soon
Who is going to do it?
Rice bowl and chopsticks in hand
I looked at their feet in the mud
And never said anything

On the eastern side of the alley
Old woman who sits at the corner
In torrents of rain, slowly sinking
Always an private smile on her face
An edge is left for bitterness
Insulates her against acquiring

The understanding heart
But once asked, it is a question
Of understanding, the language of others
The same things, by the same words
Tell her a grandiloquent statement
Bright, like neon lighting
Thoroughly she knows all the answers
Still, she asked, 'Why are you two leaving?'

THE FORTH ESTATE

Iron bell tolls black-lead days
Eyes in dark place and eyes in daylight
So many tearful eyes
But who sees the unseen devil
Does all the bad he can
To all the people he can
In all the ways that he can
As long as he can, as he does it now
As if no lives matter
Stain on a coat is unforgiven
Blood on the gun answers the question
What is written in graffiti, muttered in hell
A dying man can do nothing well
Everything that is given, is taken

But images of us are hardest to destroy
Night-scape will verify, testify
What we lose or win, is the passing moment
All goes to nothing, as dreams unborn
Street voices talk all around us
Believer of fortuneteller's art
Believer of fortune and the miracles
Fills the night till nothing left inside
But the jade of the oracles
Black was the black of darkest raven
Black-leather coat of darker covert
Blacker than the blackest heart
As statues weary of city riot
Thin black line re-drawn again
Revision by *The Inker Man* past overdue
Conjurer of happiness and sorrow
Yesterday won't forgive tomorrow
Come what will, come what way
Who records the desperate days
I found the old-world in a fountain pen
To take this indelible ink, like medicine
But the man who held the peaceful dove
Asks a hard question with a look again
Why stay here—?

AUTHOR OF GRAVES

Every morning the hearse
will pass silver shop, secret tunnel
stone bridge, lotus lake
to where wheat field meets the road

with no more warning
at the village crossroad
other than a simple barrier
falling like an exhausted arm

all will die, by and by—

So they will come here
ask her full name, here they see
what comes with ninety years
shoulder strap held up by safety pin

or how beauty fades like invisible ink
all the women who ever loved
vanished as by the mortician's touch
she was one herself—maybe

that explains everything
Louis Vuitton glamor bag
Little black Chanel dress
Cartier Tank on a too thin wrist
Her foot, in shoes of Jimmy Choo

Those were her foot-prints
some lead from the staircase
some deep in sand
some no place at all

luck fades, also, like invisible ink
how long do you reckon
out alone bare-footing

how one loss following the other
becomes the most misleading.

Orientation

We arrive as strangers in a city
Hanoi introduces herself
Her never-ending bamboo flute

Too many occidental things that day
Silver, opium, jade and gold
The tempered heat of November

Red sun rising in a sky gone cold
But she did not meet
Armando until later
She met him in The Crying Month
Two lovers on The Bridge to Heaven
The falling down of tears

All along the street the dragon
Armored, sealed, tarnish, golden
Stuff of pagodas and almond tree

With green, spring leaves after
Poems well hidden
Inside the envelope freezing air
Patriots messages, more than tearful
Winter flood fast approaching—
Corner cafe, cold coffee, wandered gaze
Take note of streets
Enter this disorientation.

The Guard House

Still the changing of the guard
outside The Cuban Embassy
one by one, one by one, one by one

the otherness has become
a suitcase: traveler, bring what you need
but now, perpetual photograph of

this negative: arms folded, legs crossed
gives away too much
travel histories, running towards or

running away, which one, Armando
you never say
by the impressions a stranger makes

behind closed green shutters
ruddy flowers in the earthenware jar
open the window before, the familiar

yesterday the studio, apartment door
wrought iron held fretwork leaves
in darker colonial patterns

to arrive in unfamiliar, other place
irrevocable, comings and goings
irreversible at passport control

the leaving of the old life, behind

now one month, later, you confess
how hollow you feel, dazed
for the first time in your life
nothing is recognizable, surrounds
unfamiliar colors

now Golden Turtle Lake, tomorrow
white birds in fields of green rice
the interminable heat—now the last piece
of Spanish nougat we share—edible paper
scorched almonds—your homeland is sweeter
impossible to recapture sweetness here.

THE SOCIAL RULES

She learned Hanoi her silk & hemp
The old houses, opium streets, the long way
Without contemplating a short-cut

There is a double vision of foreign land
The richer entire world, despite
The most dangerous avenues

But now the anchors, roots of reality
Independence and detachment mostly
People aware of one culture, one home

Exiles aware of at least two front doors
Room by room forlorn, the objects
Some were dragons and opium pipes

Small scales for weighing out the poppies
Held a bunch of misguided keys
Most doors deniably locked

Spent the entire time leading a blind man
Some roads she should never go down
Persuaded street by street, around and in-between
Now the whole city revealed, by lunchtime
Pungent lime and mint from communal tureen.

To a Friend

You are where you have been

Thirty-five streets in The Old Quarter
Beyond that, white crane birds along the river
Young green rice, waiting for sickle or scythe

A riot of rain falling from common clouds
Pattern of red lanterns on the wall inside
Poems once hidden in an almond tree

Elsewhere an outline of old ghosts
As if foretelling next season for martyrs
Blood stained paint on outside wall

Broken wine bottles on top of The Gaol
How the obvious became dangerous
Never controlled or second guessed
The height of a patriot's fall

One by one, small gestures of place
Saved by the warmth of his hand
On the small of her back
All noise and heat
Waiting for traffic lights to change
On Ly Thuong Kiet.

THE OFFERINGS

Fishing boats fall into the edge of horizon
Round boats lacquered in buffalo dung
We saw a dozen or more dolphins
Like a mighty gray congregation
Parrot-fish bright as morning rainbow
As sunrise turns the world to red
Disc of sunfish, fins catch fire
Children gathered up fish as silver
Like coins tossed for luck
Fish whose jade the sea resembles
On the cusp of sand
It is not Piha Beach
It is not Alexander Bay
But a collage of all the beaches in Asia
For a moment, think of nothing
But yellow chrysanthemums planted at low tide
Along the sand, offerings to the dead
Then the salt air tarnishes the petals
And sea-foam drags them under
Suffocated by it, washed out with talk.

Poems Of Fish

Early morning as I walked to the market
The sun was in my eyes, for a moment—

I saw *The Madonna of the Abandoned*
holding a dying man in her arms

But he was a dead fish
Every filament a small entanglement
The world a net, full of sharks

The Black Madonna smiled
And wiped her hands

Fish suffer away from water
Women say—when you cut open fish
You find poems belonging to the dead.

A Year In Shadow

The old man in the street, gray in his hair
would lift a song, long before words
come to you—completes the pain of a heart

part of what I want to tell you
is how one month became five years
with the deceptive ease of a film dissolve

for that is how the years in Hanoi appear
long sequences of dissolves
in a trick shot—lacquer bridge dissolves into rain

the French named it the spitting rain
October, wet and humid, too many promises
a different calendar, enough reasons to go

you began, to regard experiences—as if
they were about to disappear
I have begun to understand
what it means to be a foreigner

I became something, other than what I was
temporary, on some infinitely extended leave

still living in an accidental place
but am I living a real life here

when you look at crates of Beaujolais
and suitcases packed in the corner
how temporary and insignificant it all is

the days before you knew all the names
of all thirty-six streets of The Old Quarter
were happier— than the ones that came later.

ORCHARD SONG

Each apple you bite into
wears a shape of your mouth
red delicious, gala, granny smith
there is no such thing
as a bad apple between us
so we pick the worms from the pips
until the garden belongs to us
too late, said the snake, both will die
for imported apples are poisonous.

Fishing Boat

Along the beach, fish-sauce from the factories
See moonlight shadows of two brothers
Escaping in simple boats of buffalo dung

Mai, they said as they waived good-bye
Do not wait for the door to be broken down
Take your jewels and gold and leave

Take the fleet of fishing boats
And get your family away from the South
Leave behind what you cannot take

Deeds and bricks no longer matter
Under the new regime
She can't leave her sick grandfather

Soldiers come, crush her hand with a gun
Take photographs of all prisoners
Shaved heads and dark cotton uniform

Decry punishment for giving away a cigarette
Serving beef soup to soldiers
So they tortured and re-educated
Not every answer was beaten out of her body.

THE FISH SHACK

Walk along the beach
until we smell an extra strong brew
of fish sauce in the factories

Walk to the coconut thatch hut
they keep prawns in saltwater tanks
we sit, waiting for coffee

Heat coming up from the sand
and a woman squinting, as silver fish
in her net, flash a mirror of sun

I look at the beach, so years later
I will be able to see coral sand chalked
into blue arch of water

I feel fingers blindly slipping into my hand
I won't pull away;
the line to the heart, still unbroken

I am interrupted by cooking smells
the thick soup of corn and crabs
salad of banana flowers
fried fish on a plate—
I can taste it.

Envoy

The atmosphere full of brick dust
Only one Spring, saw this
Same man neighborly, he was

Smiling and shaking hands
Streets to cross Ly Thuong Kiet
To Da Tuong, no ruined luck

Past the smiling cha da tea lady
And the photocopy boys
A handclasp from an old friend
Both wear army issue socks

The manifold of the heart
There lies salvation
I saw the man walk
He wore black jacket of a spy

Under purple blossom trees
Under black tangled power lines
How a man can walk this far—
Erratically crippled.

BEYOND CHINA BEACH

The operating rooms are closed
Blood long dried inside Marble Mountain
The wounded found another way out

Lions and dragons carved deflection
Two old soldiers trace the war
Back to the demilitarized zone

In search of hideout places familiar
American boys walk grass-covered hills
Catch up to the girl who sold chewing gum

Spoke to the woman who cleaned
Army barracks, and did field-worn laundry
And was paid in detergent, boxes of Tide

The woman you passed on the street
Waited for you on the bridge
A glimpse of her face, in the taxi
But when you turned back, she had gone

Viet Cong woman sold soap powder
On the black market, that made the blast
Killed your brother

Remember the young girl who sold gum
She remembers you from years ago

How you let her climb on the tank
And sit, straddled the gun barrel

All grown up, Mai takes you up far hills
To grass-ragged demilitarized zone
Graveyard of blood, spent shells, concrete bunker

Then, just as you hear mortar fire
She will lead you back down
And make sweet coffee in her cafe.

THE NEW BLACK

Out there where orange dust settled
And defoliated the coffee bushes
Out there boy whose legs are crippled
You can give him a dollar note
But you can't buy his smile

Arabica grown in ruined soil
Espresso tells lies and secrets
Now orange toxicity haunts wasteland
Pernicious weeds refuse to grow

On a cart made of orange wood
The boy rides past on the road
The ones who know, listen to rice grow
Knee deep in the paddy fields arsenic water

Let rice simmer an hour, not more
Carrots, potatoes poisoned in the communal garden
Everything has an element of contamination
Arsenic above and below the ground

The dog at the restaurant was beaten until tender
Broth, soup, stew, braised, roasted, sausage
Ten dollars a kilo for his pedigree body
A medium size dog
Belonging to my friend.

CANON OF TIME

Tangerine is the color of jail walls
Sweet almond tree in the courtyard
Tea pots hung in high boughs

Kernels and leaves all in place
At the point of death, alive again
Patriots wrote poems of freedoms

Hid them inside crevices of bark
As old almond tree kept flowering
Praise the life of the tree, kept growing

In another time an interrogation
But the stories will be told
Broken truth and secrets, know not when

And the cold hard spotlight of gold
Words, thoughts, but that is a place never forgotten
The imported guillotine with copper bucket

That was a long time ago
Enough steel bars on each window
Paint green like wet moss

As the bony fingers holding through
Have a word to say
The soldiers in the courtyard

At play with their guns
Harsh words and harsher realities
If the speech free-running

Where starvation starts
Being the ones to tunnel underground
From one street to another

Strange mandate of old rules
In the city of citadels
The old street, the bridges

The song of the song-bird
Trapped in the French park
But, it was all one.

Faraway Birds

Shadows cast on stonewall
Columns, white like limbs
Flash of white, a songbird
Escapes the bamboo cage
White bird, white bird
Feathers blackened
In season of flame
Bird gone
Rice crop ruined
Go tell your Uncle
Famine is come—
The season of our starvation.

JOUBEN

Fruits of honey—
In the palace of your mouth
Spell-bound
There are seeds of illusion
And here between the seeds,
A simple gift of nature
That gives us pleasure
And from this
Tastes were born
Between the flowers
Perfumes were born
Between hearing and sound
Born this melody and harmony
Between your eyes and mine
The profound nature of us.

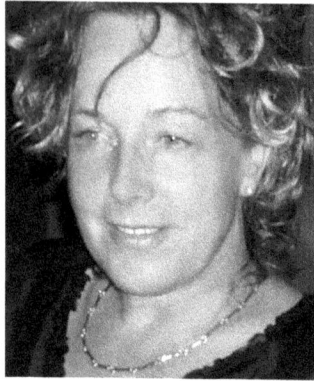

SUSAN BLANSHARD

Poet Susan Blanshard was born in Hampshire, England. She is a poet, essayist, best-selling author, revisionist poetry editor and literary critic. Her nomadic childhood and multicultural past color her writing. Susan has published selected poems such as *Fragments of the Human Heart, Quieter Histories, Poems From the Alley, Send The Raven*, and her full-length books in poetic prose include *Sheetstone*, Spuyten Duyvil, New York and *Honey in My Blood, Sleeping With The Artist*, Page Addie Press, United Kingdom. Her selected poetry and essays are published in numerous international literary magazines including The World's Literary Magazine Projected Letters, Six Bricks Press, Arabesque Magazine, Lotus International Women's Magazine, ICORN International Cities of Refuge, PEN International Women Writers' Magazine, PEN International Writers Committee The Fourth Anthology, Our Voice,

Coldnoon International Journal of Travel and Literature.

Susan Blanshard is the revisionary English poet and translations editor for seventeen translated works: poetry, literature, literary critiques, and short stories, including poetry for the winner of the 10th Cikada Prize, Sweden. Susan Blanshard is a member of PEN International Women's Writers and Asia Pacific Writers' and Translators'.

www.ingramcontent.com/pod-product-compliance
Lightning Source LLC
Chambersburg PA
CBHW050734030426
42336CB00012B/1561